STOMACH ULCER COOKBOOK FOR BEGINNERS

Quick and easy nutrient-rich recipes to manage, nourish, and soothe your gut health

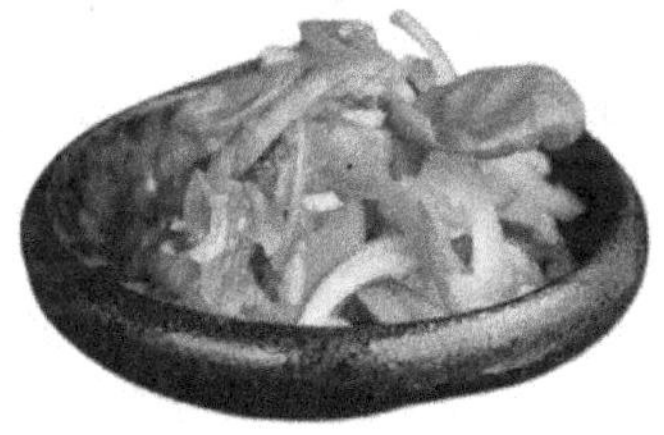

Dr. Malvin Harison

TABLE OF CONTENT

Introduction

Stomach ulcers, also known as gastric ulcers, are a prevalent gastrointestinal condition that can cause discomfort and disrupt daily life. Understanding the intricacies of stomach ulcers is crucial for effective management and improved well-being.

This introductory chapter aims to provide a comprehensive overview of stomach ulcers, their causes, symptoms, diagnosis, and the pivotal role that diet plays in their management.

Chapter 1: The overview

What is a Stomach Ulcer?

A stomach ulcer, or peptic ulcer, is a sore or hole that develops in the lining of the stomach or the first part of the small intestine, known as the duodenum. These ulcers can result from the erosion of the protective mucous layer that shields the stomach lining from digestive acids.

The most common type of stomach ulcer is caused by the bacterium Helicobacter pylori, but other factors like prolonged use of nonsteroidal anti-inflammatory drugs (NSAIDs) and excessive stomach acid production can also contribute.

Causes of Stomach Ulcers

Stomach ulcers can have various causes, and understanding these factors is vital for effective prevention and management. **The primary causes include:**

1. Helicobacter pylori Infection: A bacterial infection affecting the stomach lining.

2. NSAID Use: Prolonged use of nonsteroidal anti-inflammatory drugs like aspirin and ibuprofen.

3. Excessive Stomach Acid Production: Overproduction of gastric acids that can erode the stomach lining.

4. Smoking: Tobacco use is a known risk factor for stomach ulcers.

5. Alcohol Consumption: Excessive alcohol intake can contribute to the development of ulcers.

Symptoms and Diagnosis

Identifying the symptoms of gastric ulcers is essential for quick detection and treatment. Common symptoms include:

- **Burning Sensation**: A burning or gnawing pain in the abdomen, particularly between meals or during the night.
- **Nausea and Vomiting**; Feeling nauseous and vomiting, sometimes with the presence of blood.
- **Weight Loss**: Appetite and weight loss with no particular cause.
- **Dark, Tarry Stools**: Indicative of bleeding in the stomach.

Diagnosis often involves a combination of medical history analysis, physical examinations, and diagnostic tests such as endoscopy, blood tests, and imaging studies.

Importance of Diet in Managing Stomach Ulcers

Diet plays a pivotal role in the management and prevention of stomach ulcers. A well-balanced and stomach-friendly diet can help in reducing acidity, promoting healing, and preventing future ulcer development. In this cookbook, we will explore a variety of recipes and dietary guidelines tailored for individuals managing stomach ulcers, offering delicious and nutritious options for every meal.

Chapter 2: The Basics of a Stomach Ulcer-Friendly Diet

Stomach ulcers necessitate a mindful approach to diet for effective management and relief from symptoms. This chapter delves into the fundamental aspects of a stomach ulcer-friendly diet, providing an overview, highlighting foods to include, identifying those to avoid, and emphasizing the importance of portion control.

Overview of the Stomach Ulcer Diet

The stomach ulcer diet is designed to minimize irritation to the stomach lining, reduce acidity, and promote healing. It focuses on incorporating nutrient-rich foods that provide essential vitamins and minerals without exacerbating ulcer symptoms.

The key principles of the stomach ulcer diet include:

1. Balancing Macronutrients: Ensuring a balance of carbohydrates, proteins, and fats in each meal.

2. Emphasizing Fiber: Choosing high-fiber foods for improved digestion and gut health.

3. Incorporating Lean Proteins: Opting for lean sources of protein to minimize digestive strain.

4. Limiting Trigger Foods: Avoiding foods that can trigger or worsen ulcer symptoms.

Foods to Include

1. High-Fiber Foods: Whole grains, fruits, vegetables, and legumes provide essential fiber for digestive health.

2. Lean Proteins: Skinless poultry, fish, tofu, and legumes offer protein without excessive fat.

3. Healthy Fats: Olive oil, avocados, and nuts contribute healthy fats without causing irritation.

4. Dairy: Low-fat or fat-free dairy products can be included for calcium without the excess fat content.

Foods to Avoid

1. Spicy Foods: Spices can irritate the stomach lining, so it's advisable to avoid spicy dishes.

2. Citrus Fruits: High acidity in citrus fruits can exacerbate ulcer symptoms.

3. Tomatoes and Tomato Products: These are acidic and may cause discomfort.

4. Caffeine: Coffee, tea, and caffeinated beverages can increase stomach acid production.

5. Alcohol: Excessive alcohol intake can irritate the stomach lining and increase the risk of ulcers.

Importance of Portion Control

Controlling portion sizes is crucial for individuals with stomach ulcers. Large meals can stimulate excess stomach acid production, leading to discomfort.
Key tips for portion control include:

1. Eating Smaller, More Frequent Meals: Opting for five to six smaller meals throughout the day rather than three large ones.

2. Listening to Your Body: Paying attention to hunger and fullness cues to avoid overeating.

3. Avoiding Late-Night Eating: Consuming meals at least a few hours before bedtime to allow for digestion.

Chapter 3: Building a Balanced Plate

Creating a balanced plate is a fundamental aspect of managing stomach ulcers. This chapter explores the Plate Method tailored for stomach ulcer patients, provides insights into balancing carbohydrates, proteins, and fats, and emphasizes the importance of selecting the right fiber sources for optimal digestive health.

The Plate Method for Stomach Ulcer Patients

The Plate Method is a visual tool that simplifies meal planning and ensures a well-rounded and balanced diet. For individuals managing stomach ulcers, this method becomes particularly valuable.

The Plate Method involves dividing the plate into specific portions for different food groups:

1. Half the Plate - Vegetables: Fill half of your plate with a colorful variety of non-starchy vegetables. These provide essential vitamins, minerals, and fiber without contributing to excess acidity.

2. One-Quarter of the Plate - Lean Proteins: Reserve one-quarter of the plate for lean protein sources such as skinless poultry, fish, tofu, or legumes. These proteins aid in healing and provide necessary nutrients without causing undue digestive stress.

3. One-Quarter of the Plate - Carbohydrates: Allocate the remaining quarter of the plate to carbohydrates, focusing on whole grains like brown rice, quinoa, or whole-grain pasta.

These complex carbohydrates release energy gradually and contribute to satiety.

4. Add a Side of Healthy Fat: Include a small portion of healthy fats, such as a drizzle of olive oil on vegetables or a few slices of avocado. These fats support overall health without overloading the digestive system.

Balancing Carbohydrates, Proteins, and Fats

Achieving a harmonious balance of macronutrients is crucial for individuals with stomach ulcers. Each macronutrient plays a specific role in supporting overall health:

1. Carbohydrates: Opt for complex carbohydrates like whole grains, fruits, and vegetables.

These provide a steady release of energy and contribute essential nutrients without causing rapid spikes in blood sugar.

2. Proteins: Prioritize lean protein sources to support tissue repair and overall health. Include fish, poultry, lean meats, tofu, and legumes in your diet.

3. Fats: Choose healthy fats, such as those found in olive oil, avocados, and nuts. These fats are heart-healthy and contribute to a sense of satiety without burdening the digestive system.

Choosing the Right Fiber Sources

Fiber is a crucial component of a stomach ulcer-friendly diet as it aids digestion and promotes gut health. However, not all fiber sources are created equal. Opt for soluble fiber, found in foods like oats, barley, and fruits, as it can help soothe the digestive tract.

Insoluble fiber, found in vegetables and whole grains, should be consumed in moderation, as excessive intake may cause discomfort.

Chapter 4: Delicious Breakfast Recipes

This chapter provides practical guidance on implementing the Plate Method and achieving a balanced intake of carbohydrates, proteins, and fats while emphasizing the importance of selecting the right fiber sources for individuals managing stomach ulcers. The recipes included in subsequent chapters align with these principles, offering delicious and nourishing options.

1. Healing Smoothie Bowl

Ingredients

- 1 cup frozen mixed berries (blueberries, strawberries, raspberries)
    - 1 ripe banana
    - 1/2 cup Greek yogurt (low-fat)
    - 1 tablespoon honey
    - 1/4 cup almond milk

Preparation

- Blend all ingredients until smooth.
- Pour into a bowl and top with sliced bananas, granola, and a drizzle of honey.

2. Low-Acidity Oatmeal

Ingredients

- 1 cup old-fashioned oats
- 1 cup almond milk
- 1 tablespoon chia seeds
- 1/2 cup sliced bananas
- 1 tablespoon almond butter
- Cinnamon to taste

Preparation

- Cook oats together with almond milk.
- Stir in chia seeds, sliced bananas, and almond butter.

3. Nutritious Fruit Parfait

Ingredients

- 1 cup Greek yogurt (low-fat)
- 1/2 cup granola (low-sugar)
- 1/2 cup mixed berries (strawberries, blueberries)
- 1 tablespoon honey

Preparation

- Turn Greek yogurt and granola into layers and mixed berries bowl.
- Drizzle honey on top.

4. Baked Sweet Potato Hash

Ingredients

- 1 large sweet potato, diced
- 1/2 bell pepper, diced
- 1/2 red onion, diced
- 1 tablespoon olive oil
- 1 teaspoon smoked paprika
- Salt and pepper to taste

Preparation

- Toss sweet potato, bell pepper, and red onion with olive oil and seasonings.
- Roast in the oven until tender.

5. Banana and Almond Butter Toast

Ingredients

- 2 slices whole-grain bread
- 2 tablespoons almond butter
- 1 banana, sliced
- 1 teaspoon honey

Preparation

- Toast the bread slices.
- Spread almond butter on the toast and top with banana slices.
- Drizzle honey over the top.

6. Chia Seed Pudding with Berries

Ingredients

- 3 tablespoons chia seeds
- 1 cup almond milk
- 1/2 teaspoon vanilla extract
- 1/2 cup different berries (blueberries, raspberry, blackberry)
- 1 tablespoon shredded coconut (optional)

Preparation

- Mix chia seeds, almond milk, and vanilla extract. Refrigerate overnight.
- Top with mixed berries and shredded coconut before serving.

7. Avocado and Tomato Breakfast Wrap

Ingredients
- 1 whole-grain tortilla
- 1/2 avocado, sliced
- 1/2 cup cherry tomatoes, halved
- 2 eggs, scrambled
- Salt and pepper to taste

Preparation
- Warm the tortilla and spread avocado slices.
- Add scrambled eggs and cherry tomatoes.
- Season with salt and pepper, then wrap and enjoy.

8. Blueberry and Almond Flour Pancakes

Ingredients

- 1 cup almond flour
- 2 eggs
- 1/2 cup almond milk
- 1/2 cup fresh blueberries
- 1 teaspoon baking powder

Preparation

- Mix almond flour, eggs, almond milk, and baking powder.
- Gently fold in blueberries.
- Cook small pancakes on a non-stick skillet.

9. Quinoa Breakfast Bowl

Ingredients

- 1 cup cooked quinoa
- 1/2 cup sliced peaches

- 1/4 cup chopped almonds
- 1 tablespoon maple syrup
- 1/2 teaspoon cinnamon

Preparation

- Mix cooked quinoa with peaches, almonds, maple syrup, and cinnamon.
- Serve warm.

10. Papaya and Ginger Smoothie

Ingredients

- 1 cup papaya, diced
- 1/2 inch fresh ginger, peeled
- 1/2 cup plain kefir
- 1 tablespoon honey
- Ice cubes (optional)

Preparation

- Blend papaya, ginger, kefir, and honey until smooth.
- If desired, add ice cubes and reblend.

Chapters 5: Delicious Lunch Recipes

Here are 10 delicious, nutrient-rich, and easy-to-prepare light and nourishing lunch recipes specifically designed for stomach ulcer management. Each recipe includes natural ingredients that are gentle on the stomach and contribute to overall digestive health.

1. Grilled Chicken and Quinoa Salad

Ingredients

- 1 cup cooked quinoa
- 4 oz grilled chicken breast, sliced
- 1 cup different greens (spinach, arugula)
- 1/2 cup cherry tomatoes, halved
- 1/4 cup cucumber, sliced
- Balsamic vinaigrette dressing

Preparation

- Mix quinoa, grilled chicken, mixed greens, tomatoes, and cucumber.

- Drizzle with balsamic vinaigrette.

2. Turkey and Avocado Wrap

Ingredients
- 1 whole-grain wrap
- 3 oz turkey breast, sliced
- 1/2 avocado, sliced
- 1/4 cup shredded lettuce
- 1 tablespoon Greek yogurt (low-fat)

Preparation
- Layer turkey, avocado, and lettuce on the wrap.
- Spread Greek yogurt, then roll and secure with a toothpick.

3. Salmon and Quinoa Bowl

Ingredients
- 1 cup cooked quinoa
- 4 oz baked salmon, flaked
- 1/2 cup steamed broccoli
- 1/4 cup shredded carrots
- Lemon-tahini dressing

Preparation

- Arrange quinoa, salmon, broccoli, and carrots in a bowl.
- Drizzle with lemon-tahini dressing.

4. Vegetarian Chickpea Salad

Ingredients

- 15 oz of chickpeas, washed and drained
  - 1/2 cup of cherry tomatoes, sliced
  - 1/4 cup of red onion, finely chopped
  - 1/4 cup of feta cheese, crumbled
  - Olive oil and lemon juice dressing

Preparation

- Combine chickpeas, tomatoes, red onion, and feta cheese.
- Toss with olive oil and lemon juice dressing.

5. Miso Ginger Tofu Stir-Fry

Ingredients

- 1 cup tofu, cubed
- 1 cup mixed vegetables (broccoli, bell peppers, snap peas)
- 2 tablespoons miso paste
- 1 tablespoon low-sodium soy sauce
- 1 teaspoon fresh ginger, grated

Preparation

- Sauté tofu and mixed vegetables in a pan.
- Mix miso paste, soy sauce, and grated ginger. Pour over the stir-fry.

6. Quinoa and Black Bean Bowl

Ingredients

- 1 cup cooked quinoa
- 1/2 cup of black beans, washed, drained and rinsed
- 1/4 cup corn kernels
- 1/4 cup diced bell peppers
- Cilantro-lime dressing

Preparation

- Put together the quinoa, black beans, corn, and bell peppers.
- Drizzle with cilantro-lime dressing.

7. Spinach and Feta Stuffed Bell Peppers

Ingredients

- 2 bell peppers, halved and seeds removed
- 1 cup fresh spinach, chopped
- 1/2 cup feta cheese, crumbled
- 1/4 cup sun-dried tomatoes, chopped
- Olive oil for drizzling

Preparation

- Mix spinach, feta, and sun-dried tomatoes.
- Stuff bell peppers with the mixture and drizzle with olive oil.
- Bake until peppers are tender.

8. Lemon Herb Shrimp Salad

Ingredients

- 1 cup of shrimp, cooked and shredded
- 2 cups mixed greens (arugula, watercress)
- 1/2 cup cherry tomatoes, halved
- 1/4 cup cucumber, sliced
- Lemon-herb vinaigrette

Preparation

- Combine shrimp, mixed greens, tomatoes, and cucumber.
- Drizzle with lemon-herb vinaigrette.

9. Caprese Quinoa Salad

Ingredients

- 1 cup cooked quinoa
- 1 cup cherry tomatoes, halved
- 1/2 cup fresh mozzarella, diced
- Fresh basil leaves, chopped
- Balsamic glaze

Preparation

- Mix quinoa, tomatoes, mozzarella, and basil.
- Drizzle with balsamic glaze before serving.

10. Vegetable Lentil Soup

Ingredients

- 1 cup lentils, rinsed
- 4 cups vegetable broth
- 1 cup different vegetables (carrots, cucumber, celery, zucchini)
- 1/2 teaspoon cumin
- 1/2 teaspoon turmeric

Preparation

- Combine lentils, vegetable broth, mixed vegetables, cumin, and turmeric in a pot.
- Simmer until the lentils are tender.

Chapter 6: Delicious Dinner Recipes

Here are 10 delicious, nutrient-rich, and easy-to-prepare light and nourishing dinner recipes designed for stomach ulcer management. Each recipe includes natural ingredients that promote digestive health and contribute to overall well-being.

1. Baked Cod with Lemon and Herbs

Ingredients

- 2 cod filets
- 1 lemon, sliced
- 2 tablespoons fresh herbs (parsley, dill)
- 1 tablespoon olive oil
- Salt and pepper to taste

Preparation

- **P**reheat the oven to 400°F (200°C).
- Place cod filets on a baking sheet, top with lemon slices and herbs.

- Drizzle with olive oil, season with salt and pepper, then bake for 15-20 minutes..

2. Turkey and Vegetable Stir-Fry

Ingredients

- 1 cup turkey breast, thinly sliced
- 2 cups mixed vegetables (broccoli, bell peppers, snap peas)
- 1 tablespoon sesame oil
- 2 tablespoons low-sodium soy sauce
- 1 teaspoon fresh ginger, grated

Preparation

- Heat sesame oil in a pan, stir-fry turkey until cooked
- Add mixed vegetables and ginger, stir-fry until vegetables are tender.
- Stir in soy sauce before serving.

3. Vegetarian Chili with Beans

Ingredients

- 1 can (15 oz) kidney beans, drained
- 15 oz of black beans, washed and drained
- 1 can (15 oz) diced tomatoes
- 1 cup corn kernels
- 1 tablespoon chili powder

Preparation

- Combine beans, diced tomatoes, corn, and chili powder in a pot.
- Simmer for 20-30 minutes, stirring occasionally.

4. Grilled Veggie and Quinoa Stuffed Bell Peppers

Ingredients

- 2 bell peppers, halved and seeds removed
- 1 cup cooked quinoa
- 1 cup mixed grilled vegetables (zucchini, eggplant, bell peppers)
- 1/4 cup feta cheese, crumbled

- Olive oil for drizzling

Preparation

- Mix cooked quinoa, grilled vegetables, and feta cheese.
- Stuff bell peppers and drizzle with olive oil.
- Grill until peppers are tender.

5. Salmon and Asparagus Foil Packets

Ingredients

- 2 salmon filets
- 1 bunch asparagus, trimmed
- 1 lemon, sliced
- 2 tablespoons fresh dill, chopped
- Salt and pepper to taste.

Preparation

- Preheat the oven to 400°F (200°C).
- Place each salmon filet on a piece of foil, surrounded with asparagus.
- Top with lemon slices, dill, salt, and pepper. Seal the foil packets and bake for 15-20 minutes.

6. Mediterranean Chickpea Salad

Ingredients

- 15 oz of chickpeas, washed and drained
- 1 cup cucumber, diced
- 1 cup cherry tomatoes, halved
- 1/2 cup feta cheese, crumbled
- Kalamata olives, pitted
- Olive oil and lemon juice dressing

Preparation

- Combine chickpeas, cucumber, tomatoes, feta, and olives.
- Toss with olive oil and lemon juice dressing.

7. Stuffed Acorn Squash with Quinoa and Kale

Ingredients

- 2 corn squash, halved with seeds removed
- 1 cup cooked quinoa
- 1 cup kale, chopped
- 1/4 cup dried cranberries

- 1/4 cup pumpkin seeds

Preparation

- Roast acorn squash in the oven until tender.
- Mix quinoa, kale, cranberries, and pumpkin seeds.
- Stuff the squash of corn halves with the quinoa mixture.

8. Cauliflower and Broccoli Gratin

Ingredients

- 2 cups cauliflower florets
- 2 cups broccoli florets
- 1 cup low-fat Greek yogurt
- 1/2 cup Parmesan cheese, grated
- 1/4 cup breadcrumbs

Preparation

- Steam cauliflower and broccoli until tender.
- Mix Greek yogurt and Parmesan, fold in steamed vegetables.

- Transfer to a baking dish, sprinkle with breadcrumbs, and bake until golden.

9. Lemon Garlic Shrimp Quinoa Bowl

Ingredients

- 1 cup of cooked quinoa
- 1 cup of shrimp, peeled and deveined one
- 1 cup broccoli, steamed
- 1 tablespoon olive oil
- 2 cloves garlic, minced

Preparation

- Frizzle shrimp in olive oil with minced garlic till cooked.
- Assemble quinoa, shrimp, and steamed broccoli in a bowl.

10. Zucchini Noodles with Pesto and Cherry Tomatoes

Ingredients

- 2 medium zucchinis, spiralized
- 1 cup cherry tomatoes, halved
- 1/4 cup pine nuts
- 2 tablespoons pesto sauce
- Parmesan cheese for topping

Preparation

- Sauté zucchini noodles until tender.
- Toss with cherry tomatoes, pine nuts, and pesto sauce.
- Top with Parmesan cheese before serving.

Chapter 7: Snacks Recipes

Here are 5 delicious, nutrient-rich, and easy-to-prepare light snacks recipes designed for stomach ulcer management. Each recipe includes natural ingredients that promote digestive health and contribute to overall well-being.

1. Greek Yogurt and Berry Parfait

Ingredients

- 1 cup Greek yogurt (low-fat)
- 1/2 cup of different berries (blueberries, strawberries)
- 1 tablespoon honey
- 2 tablespoons granola (low-sugar)

Preparation

- Turn Greek yogurt, mixed berries, and granola into layer in a glass.
- Drizzle with honey before serving.

2. Cucumber and Hummus Bites

Ingredients

- 1 cucumber, sliced
- 1/4 cup hummus
- Cherry tomatoes, halved
- Fresh basil leaves

Preparation

- Spread a small amount of hummus on each cucumber slice.
- Top with cherry tomato halves and fresh basil leaves.

3. Almond and Date Energy Balls

Ingredients

- 1 cup almonds
- 1 cup dates, pitted
- 1 tablespoon chia seeds
- 1 tablespoon coconut oil
- Unsweetened shredded coconut for rolling

Preparation

- Blend almonds, dates, chia seeds, and coconut oil in a food processor until a dough forms.
- Roll into bite-sized balls and coat with shredded coconut.

4. Vegetable Sticks with Yogurt Dip

Ingredients

- Carrot and cucumber sticks
- 1/2 cup Greek yogurt (low-fat)
- 1 teaspoon lemon juice
- Fresh dill, chopped
- Salt and pepper to taste

Preparation

- Mix Greek yogurt, lemon juice, and chopped dill for the dip.
- Serve with carrot and cucumber sticks.

5. Baked Apple Chips

Ingredients

- 2 apples, thinly sliced

- 1 teaspoon cinnamon
- 1 teaspoon honey (optional)

Preparation

- Preheat the oven to 200°F (95°C).
- Fix apple slices on a cookie sheet, spray with cinnamon.
- Bake for 2-3 hours until crispy, drizzle with honey if desired.

Chapter 8: Dessert Recipes

1. Chia Seed Pudding with Mango

Ingredients

- 3 tablespoons chia seeds
- 1 cup almond milk
- 1/2 teaspoon vanilla extract
- 1 ripe mango, diced

Preparation

- Mix chia seeds, almond milk, and vanilla extract. Refrigerate overnight.
- Layer with diced mango before serving.

2. Banana and Berry Frozen Yogurt

Ingredients

- 2 ripe bananas, frozen
- 1 cup mixed berries (strawberries, blueberries)
- 1/2 cup Greek yogurt (low-fat)

- 1 tablespoon honey

Preparation

- Blend frozen bananas, mixed berries, Greek yogurt, and honey until smooth.
- Freeze for 2 hours before serving.

3. Avocado Chocolate Mousse

Ingredients

- 2 ripe avocados
- 1/4 cup cocoa powder
- 1/4 cup maple syrup
- 1 teaspoon vanilla extract

Preparation

- Ground cocoa powder, maple syrup, avocados, and vanilla extract till creamy.
- Chill before serving.

4. Coconut and Berry Parfait

Ingredients

- 1/2 cup coconut milk
- 1/2 cup Greek yogurt (low-fat)
- 1/2 cup of different berries (raspberries, blueberries, blackberry)
- 2 tablespoons shredded coconut

Preparation:

- Mix coconut milk and Greek yogurt.
- Layer with mixed berries and shredded coconut.

5. Pumpkin Spice Oat Cookies

Ingredients

- 1 cup rolled oats
- 1/2 cup pumpkin puree
- 1/4 cup maple syrup
- 1 teaspoon pumpkin spice

Preparation

- Mix rolled oats, pumpkin puree, maple syrup, and pumpkin spice.

- Drop spoonfuls onto a baking sheet and bake for 15 minutes.

Chapter 9: Beverages for Digestive Wellness

Section 1: Herbal Teas for Soothing

1. Chamomile Tea

- Traditional Uses in Digestive Health

Preparation

- Steeping Instructions

Benefit

- Anti-inflammatory Properties
- Calming Effect on Digestive System

2. Peppermint Tea

- Cooling and Soothing Qualities

Preparation

- Proper Brewing Techniques

Benefit

- Relieving Indigestion and Bloating
- Relaxation of Digestive Muscles

3. Ginger Tea

- Ancient Remedy for Digestive Issues

Preparation

- Making Fresh Ginger Tea

Benefits

- Anti-Nausea Properties
- Reduction of Stomach Discomfort

4. Licorice Root Tea

- Sweet and Soothing Herbal Infusion

Preparation

- Brewing Licorice Root Tea

Benefits

- Protection of the Stomach Lining
- Mild Laxative Effect

Section 2: Infused Water Recipes

1. Cucumber and Mint Infused Water

Ingredients
- Sliced Cucumber
- Fresh Mint Leaves
- Water

Preparation
- Combining Ingredients for Refreshing Hydration

2. Lemon and Ginger Infused Water

Ingredients
- Lemon Slices
- Fresh Ginger, Thinly Sliced
- Water

Preparation
- Infusing Water with Zesty Flavors

3. Berry Bliss Infused Water

Ingredients

- Mixed Berries (Strawberries, Blueberries)
   - Water

Preparation

- Creating a Colorful and Antioxidant-Rich Infusion

4. Citrus Splash Infused Water

Ingredients

   - Orange Slices
   - Lime Slices
   - Water

Preparation

   - Infusing Water with Citrusy Delight

Section 3: Smoothies for Gut Health

1. Banana and Spinach Smoothie

Ingredients
- Banana
- Fresh Spinach
- Greek Yogurt
- Almond Milk

Preparation
- Blending for Nutrient-Rich Smoothness

2. Pineapple and Papaya Digestive Smoothie

Ingredients
- Pineapple Chunks
- Papaya Chunks
- Coconut Water
- Chia Seeds

Preparation
- Crafting a Tropical Smoothie for Digestive Support

3. Probiotic Berry Smoothie

Ingredients

- Mixed Berries
- Kefir
- Honey

Preparation

- Incorporating Probiotics for Gut Health

4. Avocado and Kale Digestive Green Smoothie

Ingredients

- Avocado
- Kale Leaves
- Green Apple
- Coconut Water

Preparation

- Harnessing the Power of Greens for Digestive Wellness

Chapter 10: Meal Planning and Preparation Tips

Section 1: Weekly Meal Plans

Meal planning involves more than just deciding what to eat. It's about creating a consistent and balanced routine that supports your digestive system. Here, we explore the importance of meal timing, macronutrient balance, and offer tips on setting realistic goals for effective meal prep.

Importance of Consistency: Consistency in meal timing helps regulate digestive processes, promoting a more predictable and comfortable experience.

Balancing Macronutrients: A well-balanced diet includes carbohydrates, proteins, and fats. Distributing these nutrients evenly throughout the week ensures comprehensive nutrition.

Tips for Realistic Meal Prep: Setting realistic goals for meal prep is crucial. Start with manageable plans and gradually build on them as you become more comfortable with the process.

Creating a Sample Stomach Ulcer-Friendly Meal Plan

The focus is on balancing macronutrients, incorporating variety for optimal nutrient intake, and considering portion control and timing.

- **Sample Breakfast**
- Whole-grain oatmeal with sliced bananas and a sprinkle of chia seeds.
- Greek yogurt and honey with different berries.

- **Sample Lunch**
- Grilled chicken breast with quinoa and roasted vegetables.
- Spinach and feta salad with a light olive oil dressing.

- **Sample Dinner**
- Baked salmon with steamed asparagus and quinoa.
- Lentil soup with whole-grain bread.

- **Sample Snacks**
- Almond and date energy balls.
- Vegetable sticks with hummus.

Adapting Meal Plans for Personal Preferences and Dietary Needs: Not everyone has the same dietary preferences or needs. In this section, we explore how to adapt meal plans to accommodate various dietary choices, including vegetarian, vegan, gluten-free, and dairy-free options.

Vegetarian and Vegan Alternatives: Discover plant-based protein sources and creative ways to incorporate them into your meals.

Gluten-Free and Dairy-Free Alternatives: Explore delicious alternatives for those with gluten or dairy sensitivities, ensuring a diverse and satisfying diet.

Customizing for Individual Tastes and Allergies: Tailor your meal plans to suit your taste preferences and address any food allergies or sensitivities.

Section 2: Grocery Shopping for Stomach Ulcer Diet

Building a Stomach Ulcer-Friendly Grocery List: A well-prepared grocery list is the foundation of successful meal planning. In this section, we outline essential pantry staples, fresh produce selections, and other ingredients to support stomach ulcer management.

Essential Pantry Staples: Stock your pantry with whole grains, lean proteins, healthy fats, and legumes for a well-rounded diet.

Fresh Produce and Seasonal Choices: Explore the optimal fruits and vegetables that contribute to digestive health and add variety to your meals.

Navigating the Grocery Store with Digestive Wellness in Mind: Not all foods are created equal when it comes to digestive wellness. Learn to make strategic choices, such as opting for whole foods over processed options and reading labels to identify potential irritants.

Choosing Whole Foods: Selecting minimally processed foods provides a higher nutritional value and is generally gentler on the digestive system.

Reading Labels for Hidden Irritants: Become adept at deciphering food labels to identify ingredients that might trigger stomach discomfort.

Meal Prep Ingredients: Consider the balance between convenience and freshness when choosing ingredients for your meal preparation.

Smart Shopping Habits for Stomach Ulcer Diet Success: Smart shopping involves more than just picking items off the shelf. In this section, discover the importance of meal prep containers, creating and sticking to a shopping list, and choosing high-quality ingredients for a successful stomach ulcer diet.

Meal Prep Containers and Storage Solutions: Invest in containers that support your meal preparation routine and keep your food fresh.

Making a Shopping List and Sticking to It: A well-organized shopping list helps you stay focused, save time, and stick to your dietary goals.

Choosing High-Quality Ingredients: Prioritize the quality of your ingredients to enhance the nutritional value and digestive benefits of your meals.

Section 3: Cooking Techniques for Digestive Comfort

Steaming and Poaching: Retain the nutritional value of your ingredients by incorporating gentle cooking methods like steaming and poaching.

Grilling and Roasting Tips: Enhance the flavor of your meals with grilling and roasting while ensuring they remain gentle on your digestive system.

Herbs and Spices for Flavor Without Irritation: Discover the world of digestive-friendly seasonings. Learn about herbs and spices that add depth to your meals without causing irritation.

Find a balance in flavor profiles, reducing reliance on salt and strong spices.

Introduction to Digestive-Friendly Seasonings: Explore herbs and spices known for their digestive benefits and pleasant flavors.

Balancing Flavor Profiles: Create well-rounded and flavorful dishes by combining various herbs and spices thoughtfully.

Reducing Reliance on Salt and Strong Spices: Learn how to cut back on salt and strong spices, opting for more gentle alternatives without sacrificing taste.

Portion Control and Mindful Eating: Portion control is a critical aspect of digestive wellness.

In this section, we explore the benefits of managing portion sizes and implementing mindful eating habits to enhance digestive satisfaction.

Benefits of Portion Control: Discover how controlling portion sizes can minimize stomach distress and improve overall well-being.

Implementing Mindful Eating Habits: Learn how to be present and mindful during meals, promoting a healthier relationship with food.

Chapter 11: Beyond the Kitchen - Lifestyle Tips for Managing Stomach Ulcers

Stress Management Strategies

Living with stomach ulcers can be challenging, and stress is known to exacerbate digestive issues. In this section, we'll explore effective stress management strategies to help you maintain a calm and balanced lifestyle.

1. Mindfulness Meditation
 Benefits
   - Stress Reduction
   - Improved Emotional Well-being
 Practice
   - Find a quiet space, focus on your breath, and let go of racing thoughts.

2. Yoga and Gentle Exercise

Benefits

- Physical and Mental Relaxation
- Improved Digestion

Practice

- Explore yoga poses and gentle exercises that promote relaxation.

3. Breathing Exercises

Benefits

- Calming the Nervous System
- Enhancing Focus

Practice

- Try deep breathing exercises to reduce stress and promote a sense of calm.

The Role of Exercise in Digestive Health

Exercise is not only beneficial for your overall health but can also positively impact your digestive system. In this section, we'll explore how regular physical activity contributes to digestive wellness.

1. Improving Gut Motility

Benefits

- Enhanced Digestive Function
- Reduced Constipation

Exercise

- Engage in activities like brisk walking or jogging.

2. Reducing Stress-Induced Digestive Issues

Benefits

- Stress Reduction
- Prevention of Stress-Related Ulcer Flare-ups

Exercise

- Add exercises like cycling and swimming into your schedules.

3. Maintaining a Healthy Weight
Benefits

- Balanced Digestive System
- Reduced Pressure on the Stomach

Exercise

Adequate Sleep for Healing

Quality sleep is essential for overall health and plays a crucial role in the healing process. In this section, we'll explore the connection between sleep and digestive healing.

1. Promoting Tissue Repair
Benefits
- Cellular Regeneration
- Stomach Lining Repair

Sleep Hygiene
- Create a good sleep schedule and establish a calming bedtime routine.

2. Balancing Hormones
Benefits
- Hormonal Regulation
- Reduced Stress Hormones

Sleep Hygiene:
- Create a comfortable sleep environment, free from distractions.

3. Enhancing Overall Well-being
 Benefits
   - Improved Mood
   - Mental Clarity
Sleep Hygiene
   - Reduce screen time prior to bed and practice relaxation techniques.

Conclusion

Maintaining a stomach ulcer-friendly lifestyle goes beyond what you eat. By incorporating stress management strategies, regular exercise, and prioritizing adequate sleep, you create a holistic approach to managing stomach ulcers. Consistency in these lifestyle factors contributes not only to digestive health but also to your overall well-being.

As we conclude this guide, remember that managing stomach ulcers is a journey, and each individual may find a unique balance that works best for them. Pay attention to your body's signals, be mindful of lifestyle choices, and seek support from healthcare professionals when needed. May your journey to digestive wellness be filled with vitality and comfort.